Tashirat Recipe Manual

Tashirat Recipe Manual

By
Tashirat staff

Tashirat Recipe Manual

Tashirat Learning Center, Tepoztlan, Mexico
© 2014 by Tashirat Staff

For information address:
www.Tashirat.com

tashiratmail@gmail.com

The medical and health procedures in this book are based on the research, training and personal experience of the author. As each one of us and each situation is unique, the reader is urged to check with a qualified health professional when in doubt, before applying any procedure, and preferably to work under his / her supervision.

ISBN: 978-1-304-72223-2 (Pbk)

Cover Photo by Chris Mezera
Back Photo by Thyesha Arian

Note to the Reader

This book is replete with knowledge that takes the reader's cosmic consciousness for granted. In addition, it can only be understood if the following books by Artimia Arian are read in the order presented:

Cosmic Reawakening

Vibrational Nutrition

A Cosmic Understanding of Disease and Cure

Timeless Spiritual Teachings

Inspirational Quotes for the New Era

Essential Teachings for the New Era

Spiritual Vision for the New Era

For supplemental information please also read:

To Life!

Chakra Recipe Guide

The Tashirat Recipe Manual

For convenience, the masculine has been utilized not the feminine and they have not been used alternately as was done in some of my other books. No preference of sex is intended.

In Truth, Love and Life,
Artimia Arian

Contents

Introduction

Since opening the Tashirat Orphanage for abandoned and abused children in 2003, we have constantly had to revamp our kitchen to keep our children happy and satisfied with their food as well as healthy. Although prior to the orphanage we had years of experience creating healthy and appetizing dishes for ourselves and to teach students in our Learning Center, none of this has been as challenging as keeping our kids' cuisine always new and exciting for them. The following recipe manual is the result of the creativity and effort of the Tashirat staff members to rise to this challenge. The recipes included in this manual are the personal favorites of our children and staff.

We encourage you to use this book to get started, but to rely on your own taste and creativity to develop your own healthy favorites too. The purpose of this manual is to give you many different options to choose from, while adhereing to the basic principles of correct food combining, something we found it was hard to come by in many other vegetarian cook books. We know that when changing one's diet (eliminating unhealthy staples such as meat, sugar, refined foods and dairy) one is often left wondering, "what can I eat?!"

This recipe book provides recipes from Chakra 2 proteins (such as eggs and legumes) to Chakra 5 raw food dishes, although the focus is mostly on Chakra 2, 3 and 4 dishes. Whatever your diet, always include green salads, lightly steamed and/or raw vegetables as accompanionment to your main dish for a healthy and balanced vegetarian diet. In most cases, we have listed the recipes for main dishes, salads and dressings separately, so feel free to mix and match according to your taste! Just be careful to adhere to proper food combining guidelines, as outlined in our previous nutrition books.

Most of the recipes in this manual are not included in our three previous books, The Chakra Recipe Guide, To Life! and Simply Simple (located at the back of Yoga, Path of Life). The Chakra Recipe Guide and To Life! provide the dietary and nutritional knowledge you will need to eat well and feel well, whatever your current diet, for example: how to combine foods properly, why and when we should eliminate certain foods from the diet, substitutions for those foods, and guidelines on how to make a complete transition to the highest vibration, most nutritious vegan and raw diet, including recipes. Simply Simple is a completely raw recipe guide. Therefore, for a complete transitional cuisine and nutritional guidelines, you should use all four books as a reference.

Some of the following recipes do not follow the food combining guidelines strictly e.g. several dessert recipes mix protein and fruit, some of the complex carbohydrates dishes include protein (dairy) or several proteins mixed in the same dish, all of which can compromise digestion for some, and in general delays digestion time and puts a strain on the body, although you may not notice any acute adverse effects. Although our staff members adhere strictly to the food combination guidelines, we are not very strict with our older children as long as such mixes do not overtly affect them. Please refrain from making bad combinations if you have a sensitive / weak digestión or are unwell. The dairy included in some of the complex carbohydrate dishes can easily be omitted or substituted for avocado, whipped avocado "cream" or guacamole (avocado also digests as a carbohydrate, thus it combines well with the complex carbohydrates/starches). Most of the protein recipes are very well combined and there are many properly combined sweet treat ideas to choose from as well.

As in our previous recipe books, we haven't given specific quantities for many of the recipes. We have done this in an effort to simplify and leave room for you to personalize your dishes as much as possible. Food preparation is such a "feel", and each person has different tastes, so we have left it up to you, as the cook, to add as much or as little of certain ingredients as you would like. Experiment, have fun and please share with us any great new recipes you invent!

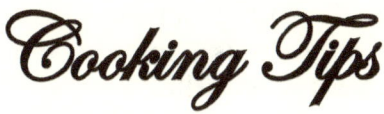

Cooking Tips

The best scrambled eggs
For fluffy scrambled eggs, always beat eggs in blender with tiny bit of water (or unsweetened soy milk or cow's milk) before cooking.

Keep food from sticking to the pan, without frying
Drizzle a few drops of oil in the pan, then wipe clean with a tissue before cooking. Use Teflon (non-stick) pans. NEVER fry food in oil (it's frying when you hear that sizzling sound). If necessary, add olive oil right after removing food from the stove or oven, cover and let sit for a few minutes to add flavor. Always heat the pan (until water sizzles immedly when dropped on the pan) before cooking burgers, eggs or patties, so they don't stick.

How to cook patties
Cook all patties (tortas) on <u>low heat</u> so they dry all the way through before the outside starts to burn. Flip patties once they are fully dried around the edges and bottom. If you try to flip too soon, they will fall apart. These instructions are also helpful for making "fried" eggs.

Salsas and Chiles
*Cooking **peppers and tomatoes** -* Cook red peppers, tomatoes, green tomatoes etc. in a bit of soy sauce and water until the skin slips off easily. Remove the skins if desired or blend as is

Chopped salsas - When making chopped salsas (e.g. pico de gallo), be sure to chop the ingredients very finely so the flavors combine. Also, by adding a tiny bit of water or lemon and olive oil, the flavors are enhanced.

Try different chiles - Use different types of chiles to change the flavor of your standard red salsa. Some good options to try are: chile de arbol (dry roast with garlic), serrano, the small green chile and jalapeno, the larger green chile (sauté fresh with onion and garlic), habanero, a yellow or orange bulbous chile (sauté fresh, but only for those who really like it spicy!)

Dried chiles - Remove the seeds and vein from the chile guajillo, ancho or pasilla after soaking the chiles in warm water until softened. Take the seeds out of the chile de arbol also after toasting, or it will be very spicy! Don't touch the seeds with your bare fingers, its hard to remove the chiles "burn" even after washing thorougly.

Non-spicy chile: How to us just for flavor - Before using serrano chiles in a dish, roll on a table to enhance their flavor. Put one or two whole chiles into a stew, soup or pot of beans during cooking to add flavor without making them spicy.

Subtle Seasoning With Garlic and Onion
Give subtle flavor to broth or refried beans by sautéing garlic and onion in the same pan you later use to heat beans or a tomato broth in, without rinsing in between. Use the onion or garlic in a salsa or discard.

Soups
Add great flavor#1 - Submerging a few sprigs of cilantro (minus the root) into the simmering broth, then turn off the heat and leave submerged for five minutes before serving.

Add great flavor#2 - Saute onions in a pan until transparent, then add the broth spices, water and vegetables and cook.

Non-dairy soup or topping - To make a non-dairy soup, or well combined complex carbohydrate topping – blend avo with a tiny pinch of salt and lemon (optional) until smooth and put on top of the soup as a cream (could also garnish with pico de gallo).

Vegetables

Carrots - Peel carrots before serving in raw salads or steaming only if their skin is blemished. It is unnecessary to peel carrots before grating unless they look unfresh. The skin of the carrot contains a large amount of its vitamins, so leave it on if they're very fresh. Buy small carrots as they are usually tenderer, juicier and have cleaner skin.

Cucumbers - Pick the freshest cucumbers by checking that they are very hard all the way to the ends. The tasier, sweeter cucumbers are the narrower variety. Often people, children especially, are turned away from vegetables because they haven't had a freash one!

Tomatoes - If you can't get fresh, unwaxed tomatoes, buy the hydroponic round variety which are mostly unwaxed. The wax peserves the fruit but has a lot of chemicals and changes the taste. Only fresh, good quality produce tastes good.

Preparation of legumes

Soak the legumes 12 hours, sprout for 12 hours, then cook as little as possible, preferably steam (lentils 5-10 minutes and chickpeas 10 -15 minutes) before using in any dish. This makes them much easier to digest, even for those with weak digestion. It also facilitates the assimilation of their nutrients in the process of digestion, because they are sprouted.

If a dish doesn't turn out well, revamp it!
Try to doctor it up or serve it in a different way before just throwing it out. Our sunflower seed burgers were the result of a failed attempt at mock-tuna salad one day. Our baked lentil dish was the result of a large quantity of leftover lentil soup that didn't

go over well with the kids one day and became a total success the next!

Easy blender cleaning
Fill the blender ½ full with water and some dishwashing soap, and blend for a minute or so, then rinse by hand. For very sticky foods, blend longer.

Appliance cleaning and stain removal
Soak your juicer parts, blender pitcher or any other stained kitchen appliance parts in water mixed with chlorine bleach. Wash thoroughtly before using for food preparation again.

Proteins

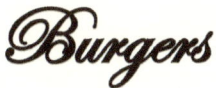

Burgers

Seed or Nut Burgers:

Sunflower seed burgers
Blend about 1 lb of raw sunflower seeds, ½ an onion, a sprig of cilantro and 1 celery stalk in the food processor. Form patties and slowly brown both sides on low heat.

Sesame seed burgers
Toast about 1 lb of sesame seeds and blend with a little water and garlic. Grate 3 zucchinis and 3 carrots. Chop a bit of onion and cilantro. Mix in a bowl. Form patties and slowly brown both sides on low heat.

Almond Meal burgers
Use the strained off fiber left over from making almond milk. Mix with grated carrot and celery, diced red pepper, and onion (optional). Form patties and slowly brown both sides on low heat. Optional: add mushroom.

Legume burgers:

Garbanzo burgers
Make hummus (follow the hummus recipe but omit the oil or the burgers will fry), form into burgers, add chopped onion, cilantro or chipotle chile.

Sprouted lentil burgers
Sprout the lentils, chop red pepper, onion and cilantros finely, blend the lentils in the food processor with a few carrots, cumin and curry. Mix everything together.

Cooked lentil burgers

Cook lentils until all the excess water is cooked off, mash the lentils into a paste and add grated vegetables such as carrot, zucchini, chopped onions and cilantro. Form into patties and brown both sides on low heat.

Soy-based burgers:

Soy meat burger

This recipe mixes two proteins so it is not recommended for those with weak digestions, but it's a great alternative to hamburgers. Mix boiled soy meat (the pre-flavored kind with spices is tastiest) with beaten eggs and chopped onion, then cook the batter in patties.

Tofu burger

Make tofunesa (the almonds should be 1/3 unsoaked and 2/3 soaked) making sure to blend in a food processor, not blender so as to refrain from using more water than absolutely necessary or batter will not be thick enough to make burgers. If that happens, you can always make tofunesa or a tofu scramble (see recipes in tofu section).

Okara (soy bean fiber) burger

Use the fiber left over from making soymilk. Press as much of the milk out of the leftover fiber as you can in a fine strainer or cheese cloth. Then mix with onion and cilantro or chipotle and red pepper, or any herbs you choose. Form patties and slowly brown both sides over low heat.

Egg-based burgers:

Egg, zucchini, and cheese burger
Whip eggs in the blender, mix with grated zucchini and pour into the pan in the form of large cookie sized circles. Cover the pan with a lid for a few minutes, and then flip patties and cook for another 2 minutes. (Optional: add a slice or spinkle of cheese, cover, and cook for about 1 more minute before serving).

Eggs and mixed veggie burger
This is a variation of the first egg burger recipe. Veggie combos could be:
Mushroom, red pepper and onion
Onion and spinach
Peas and brocoli
Grated carrot and zucccini

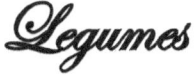

Legumes

Chickpeas in green chile
Prepare according to Cooking Tips "Preparation of lentils and chickpeas", cooking for 5 minutes only. Prepare a green salsa (see Salsas) and cook the chickpeas for another 10 minutes in the salsa with 1 whole clove of garlic, a whole serrano pepper slit on the sides. Turn off and add 1 tsp. olive oil. Let sit 15 minutes as the flavors combine.

Chickpeas Mexican style
Prepare chickpeas as in Cooking Tips, cooking for the full 15 minutes. Let cool for 10 minutes and then mix with pico de gallo (see Salsas).

Hummus

Soak, cook and blend garbanzos with sautéed garlic and onion, tahini, oil and lemon until very smooth. About 4 – 6 lemons are used in each big food processor batch. Saute onion and garlic very well so the flavor isn't too strong. You can also add sautéed red bell pepper or chipotle chile.

Hummus tacos or sopes

Heat corn tortillas, or sopes and top with hummus and grated cheese and marinated chile slices or "rajas". Serve with your salsa of choice, chopped lettuce, sliced or grated radish and chopped cilantro.

Easy lentil dahl

Boil about 1 lb of lentils and strain. Sautee 1 diced onion, garlic, and 3 diced tomatoes and mix with lentils, finely chopped cilantro and curry powder or garam masala.

Lentil bake

Bake cooked lentils with thick tomato sauce and cheese on top

Lentil soup

Pan sear about diced tomatoes and ½ of a diced onion, add sprouted lentils and boil until soft. Add ½ tsp cumin and a big sprig of finely chopped cilantro.
Serve with olive oil, sour cream and grated cheese (optional).

Blended lentil soup

Blend lentil soup (refer to recipe above) with more pan seared tomato and garlic.

White beans in chili guallilo, tomato, cilantro broth

Boil about 1 lb of beans. Blend about 6 tomatoes, 6 guallilo peppers, garlic, onion and strain to make a sauce. Add sauce and a sprig of cilantro to the strained beans and cook an additional 10-15 minutes.

Black bean soup
Boil about 1 lb of black beans with 1 diced onion and some epazote (optional), and saute ¼ lb chile poblano peppers with soy sauce. Serve beans with cream and the sauteed peppers, cut into srtips.

Refried black or bayo beans
Cook black beans as above, strain and blend with some of their broth until a smooth and thick past is formed. Serve on tostadas, with tortillas or as is, with pico de gallo and grated cheese and cream (dairy optional).

Lima bean soup
Boil about 1lb. of lima beans. Sautee ½ diced onion, garlic, and about 5 tomatoes. Add finely chopped mint and all other ingredientes to the beans.

Fava bean (habas) salad
Boil the fresh shelled beans until tender, adding salt at the end of the cooking time. Let sit until very sofr, then strain and mix with chopped cilantro, onion, and tomato, a little olive oil, lemon and sea salt.

Fava bean paste
Soak dried (yellow) fava beans overnight. Boil until soft and mushy. Blend with sautéed onion in a food processor until forms a thick paste, like hummus. Add salt and oil as desired.

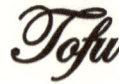
Tofu

Stir fry
Cut tofu in small cubes and brown in a Teflon pan. Cut all vegetables in little pieces and stir fry in a separate pan. Once the tofu is browned, add to the stir fry and season.

Tofunesa dip
Blend uncooked tofu with a little bit of chipotle pepper, onion and garlic, a pinch of oregano and about 1/5 a red bell pepper per person. The dip should be a light salmon color. Be careful not to overdo it with any of the ingredients, especially the oregano – taste as you prepare!

Tofu burger or scramble
See Soy-based burgers in the burgers Protein section.

Tofu crumble
Steam very finely diced vegetables. Crumble tofu by hand and cook in a Teflon pan with soy sauce. Mix the vegetables with the tofu and add olive oil.
Variation: cook as above with the addditon of hot sauce.

Mexican style tofu
Cut tofu in small cubes and brown in a Telfon pan. Add diced onion and tomatoes when the tofu is nearly ready and leave to cook until the tomatoes and oinion are sautéed.

Pan browned tofu
Cut thin strips of tofu, sprinkle or dip in soy sauce and brown on a Teflon pan. Once browned, serve as is or cover with a mild garlic and tomato sauce and continue to heat on a low flame. These can also be served with barbecue sauce.

Baked tofu
Bake thinly sliced tofu (or whole blocks) in the oven with curry and soy sauce.

Tofu lasagna
Form layers of thinly sliced zucchini, tomato sauce and crumbled browned tofu in an oven pan and bake until the zucchini is cooked. Cover with cheese before baking if desired.

Miso soup
Brown cubed tofu in Teflón pan with soy sauce. Boil water and add bowned tofu, sauteed onions, finely cubed carrots, shallots and peas. Once the vegetables have cooked, turn off the soup and add miso paste to the hot broth, stirring until it dissolves.

Chayote almond soup
Steam and blend 2 chayotes with a handful of soaked almonds or pecans, and sea salt. Optional: add garlic and parley. Pan brown small cubes of tofu and add the pureed soup.

Tofu tomato soup
Saute tomatoes in a pan, whole, until their skins slide off. Then blend with a little piece of garlic (optional) and add crumbled pan browned tofu and steamed vegetables.

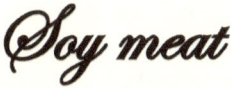

Soy meat in tomato sauce
Sauté onion, garlic, tomatoes and blend. Add dry soy meat to the sauce and boil until the soy meat has absorbed all the sauce.

"Chorizo" or Mexican style spicy ground sausage

Cook dry soy meat in salsa guajillo in a pan until all the sauce has cooked off.

Soy meat "escabeche" or warm vinaigrette salad

Boil the soy meat in water with aromatic herbs and mix with finely diced steamed vegetables, apple cider vinager, olive oil and sea salt. Add oregano (optional)

Soy meat ceviche

Boil strain and drain soy meat. Press out all excess water. Mix with pico de gallo (diced tomato, onion, cilantro and chile verde), salt and a little olive oil.

Italian style ground sausage

Make the soy meat in tomato sauce (make sure it was boiled in the least amount of sauce possible so it can be dried out). Add a few eggs, and spices such as cumin, thyme, etc. to the soy meat and cook in a pan.

Tostadas

Serve soy meat "chorizo" on baked tostadas (these are tortillas that have been oiled and baked in oven) with cream, cheese, diced tomato, lettuce, onion, and serrano chile (optional).

Taco salad

Serve soy meat "chorizo" mixed into a salad (lettuce, spinach, tomato, cucumber, grated carrot) with grated cheese or sliced soft white cheese (panela) and tortillas.

Soy meat burgers

See Soy-based burgers in the Burgers-Protein section

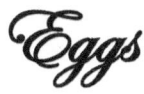

Eggs

Spinach zucchini egg patties
Finely chop spinach, onion and calabaza and mix with beaten eggs. Use a big serving spoon to pour pancake size patties onto the pan. Cook the same as pancakes.

Mexican style eggs
Eggs scrambled with sautéed diced tomatoes and onions, chile serrano optional.

Chile con huevo
Heat a pot of tomato broth, made of pan-seared tomatoes blended with a small piece of chile, garlic and onion. Then add fluffy scambled eggs and a sprig of cilantro.

"Fried" eggs
Break whole eggs into a very lightly preoiled Teflon pan without breaking the yoke. Flip once. Serve on a corn tortilla (optional) and top with pico de gallo, chopped lettuce and salsa, with steamed chayote (optional) and jicama on the side.

Scambled eggs with vegetables
Lightly steam greenbeans or zuchinni (chopped or grated) and mix into scambled eggs while cooking.

Hard-boiled egg tacos
Hard-boiled eggs, salad and salsa of choice rolled into a tortilla (recommended: pico de gallo with grated veggies, chopped letttuce, topped with a salsa or chile piquin).

Egg dipped cauliflower or broccoli florets
Beat egg whites separately until fluffy, then mix in the yolks. Dip chunks of steamed cauliflower into the batter and brown in Teflón

pan. Serve with or in a tomato sauce, with chopped raw onion (and green chile, optional) that has been marinated for at least 10 minutes in lemon juice.

Omelette
Pour eggs into a Teflon pan (like a big pancake). Fill with cheese, sautéed onion, tomatoes and spinach or any other vegetables of choice and fold in half once you are able to flip.

Alfalfa sprout tortas
Dip handfuls of sprouts into blended egg, cook in a pan in the form of patties. Once you cook one side, add a little more egg to the top (raw side) with a spoon right before flipping. Serve the tortas in thick tomato sauce.

Savory Crepes
Blend eggs with wheat germ to make a batter (the eggs will thicken with the wheat germ but still run off the spoon). Make thin pancakes and fill with sautéed vegetables or mushrooms.

Egg salad
Dice boiled eggs, add cubed steamed vegetables such as string beans, chayote, and zucchini and mix with paprika or cayenne and soy mayonnaise or sour cream.

Egg n' cheese pancakes
Blend eggs, a little wheat germ and grated cheese until fluffy. Make small pancakes and serve with ketchup, lettuce and onion in rings (optional) on top.

Dairy dishes

*We rarely use milk and/or cheese as the main base of a dish, as they are very mucous-forming. We prefer to use milk products as a topping, just to make dishe look especially appetizing. Here are a few recipes that use more than the usual sprinkle or drizzle of cheese and cream. When coming up with your own dairy dishes, try to use the soft, mild, white cheeses, like ricotta, cottage cheese, and panela, as they are healthier than the hard, sharp, yellow cheeses. Yogurt is a healthier substitute for sour cream.

Zuchinni or poblano peppers stuffed with ricotta cheese or beans
Cut a slit in the side of the peppers and remove the seeds. Roast chilis directly on the stove (in the flame). Remove from the flame and place in a plastic bag once the skin is scorched. Peel skin off of chilis once they have been in the bag for 10 minutes. Steam the zuchinnis lightly and remove the insides. Stuff vegetables with ricotta cheese or beans and add tomato sauce.

Chayotes in cream sauce
Peel and slice chayotes in roundsand steam. Beat cream into a tomato sauce, and serve chayotes bathed in a generous helping of it. Variation: melt cheese on top.

Steamed vegetables with melted cheese and toasted sesame seed
Steam a variety of vegetables, transfer to a pan and sprinkle with cheese. Cover the pan and cook until cheese is melted. Add toasted sesame before serving.

Tomato salad with panela cheese

Dice tomates or use whole cherry tomatoes combined with cubes of panela cheese, minced fresh basil and olive oil.

Complex Carbohydrate
Starches

*The following recipes contain starches, so *ideally* should not be mixed with proteins such as cheese. If your digestion is sensitive or you are unwell please omit the dairy products (cream and cheese) from the following recipes, and use avocado instead.

Tortilla dishes

Enfrijoladas
Boil black beans with diced onion, and a chile serrano (a whole chile that is removed after cooking). Blend the beans in a little of their broth, with a little bit of olive oil and sauteed onion. Dip tortillas one by one, covering both sides with the bean paste, and serve with pico de gallo, shredded lettuce, poblano peppers, lettuce, cream and cheese on top.

Enchiladas
Toast and roll torillas with filling of choice (steamed vegetables, panela cheese, or sautéed mushrooms or all three) and cover liberally with either red or green salsa. Serve with grated cheese and chopped lettuce and onion.

Chilequiles
Slice tortillas (like mini pizza slices) and toast in a pan or leave in the sun to harden. Cook in a pan with layers of salsa of choice. Serve with lettuce, cream and cheese.

Tacos
Make tacos out of just about anything wrapped in a fresh corn tortilla!
Some suggestions are:
Avocado mashed with a little sea salt
Rice and vegetables
Mashed potatoes

Soy meat
Eggs
Beans
Vegetables (grated) with cheese or avocado slices
Different kinds of mushrooms sautéed with onions

Quesadillas

These are very similar to tacos only that they invariably contain melted cheese and they can also be made with two tortillas melted together, instead of one folded tortilla. Put cheese and whatever else from the above list between two tortillas and heat in a covered pan, "comal" or skillet, flipping once.

Pita bread and Whole wheat rolls

Pita pocket sandwich

Toast whole-wheat pita bread and open it on one side. Stuff the pita bread with grated raw or stir-fried vegetables, or guacamole with shredded lettuce, carrot etc.

Pita pizza

Toast whole-wheat pita bread and add toppings of choice (spinach, olives, bell peppers, tomatoes, onion, mushrooms etc.), tomato sauce with Italian herbs and melted cheese. Toast bread very well so it is less starchy and therefore easier to digest with protein.

Pita chips

Cut pita breads into triangles, like you would a pie, then bake in an oven, or on the stove in a pan, until dry and crispy. Serve with avocado dip, or with soups or salads.

Whole wheat bun sandwich

Spread a whole wheat roll with refried beans, or a a fried egg and a slice of panela cheese.This is an easy, typical Mexican school snack, but not a good food combination. A much healthier alternative would be avocado slices, lettuce and tomato, but be careful not to slice the avocado more than an hour before it will be eaten as it turns brown.

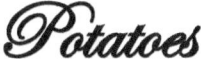

Potatoes

French fries
Slice into thick fries, then steam potatoes or sweet potatoes until half cooked, then transfer to an oiled cookie sheet or baking pan and continue cooking in the oven until brown and crispy. May need turning over to crisp on both sides is desired. Serve with fructose sweetened ketchup.

Baked potatoes
Wash and gently massage whole potatoes with a little bit of olive oil, and then bake. Or wrap each potato in tin foil and bake. Cut down the center and top with herbs, salt and olive oil, butter, cream or cheese, or for better food combining, avocado. Serve with broccoli or other steamed vegetables and or raw salad as desired.

Mashed potatoes
 Boil whole potatoes and mash with a fork or blend in a food processor with butter until creamy.

Potatoes with vegetarian ham
This is not a very good mix but is a favorite treat for our older kids. Boil the potatoes, peel and cut into medium sized cubes. Saute the cubes in a pan with vegetarian ham (also cut in squares) until the potato cubes are browned.

Potato patties

Boil potatoes, then mash them with a fork not with a food processor, while adding the yolk of an egg (per 3 potatoes). Form patties with the potato-egg mash, adding finely chopped onion if desired. Before cooking each patty, lightly coat with the egg white by dipping your hands in the white and gently handling the patty before transferring to the pan.

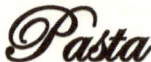

Spaghetti
Boil whole wheat, spinach or spelt spaghetti as directed on the package. Mix with finely chopped steamed vegetables of choice and serve topped with tomato sauce, Italian herbs and cream or cheese. We add a lot of steamed vegetables with the spaghetti such as broccoli, zucchini, carrot, chayote, peas, spinach etc.

Variation1: Skip the tomato sauce and just drizzle the pasta and vegetables with a dressing of sauteed garlic blended with olive oil and fresh basil.
Variation 2: While the pasta is still hot, add butter and mix thoroughly until melted.
Variation 3: Cover the pasta and vegetables in a tomato sauce mixed with cream.

Lasagna
Same as the tofu dish made of zucchini "noodles" but with real pasta. Cook pasta and make layers of pasta, sauce and ricotta cheese or tofu, Finishing with a layer of cheese on top.

Tomato noodle soup
Make a tomato soup base with pan seared tomatoes and a little garlic or onion. Then add precooked elbow or shell shaped noodles.

Vegetable noodle soup

Boil finely chopped herbs and vegetables in pure water for about 15 minutes, and then turn over the heat, cover and let sit for anoth 15 minutes. Add some butter and about a spoon of cream per liter of water and the precooked noodles, and serve. If you prefer to omit the dairy, add mashed or blended avocado and oil instead of butter and cream.

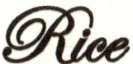

Mexican rice

Cook rice, adding tomato sauce and steamed peas and fined cubed steamed carrots at the end. Top with olive oil, herbs and salsa of choice. Other vegetable options: zucchini, broccoli, chayote, green beans.

Rice stir-fry

Cook rice and mix into a stir-fry of vegetables that have been sautéed in soy sauce. Vegetable suggestions: mung bean sprouts, zucchini, broccoli and carrot.

Zucchini rice

Cook rice and mix with raw shredded zucchini and carrot. Serve with avocado or a blended avocado and tomatillo salsa.

Sushi

Fill Nori sheets with a layer of brown rice (stir it during cooking, then let to cool, without stirring, so it "gels"), sprouts, thin carrot and cucumber sticks and avocado slices. Roll and cut into bite-size pieces. Serve with chopped ginger and garlic marinated in soy sauce, avocado dressing, or lemon, oil and soy sauce.

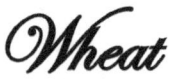

Taboule

Soak or boil cracked wheat. Add cubed tomatoes, finely diced onion and cucumber, finely chopped mint and parsley. Top with lemon, olive oil and salt. Serve with avocado and lettuce

Mushroom and Wheat Pozole (a variation of the traditional Mexican Pozole)

Boil wheat berries and add chopped mushrooms. Blend garlic and guallilo peppers in water, strain and add to soup. Serve with finely diced onion and radish. Mix in a little bit of orégano.

Crepes

Blend eggs with wheat germ. Use more wheat germ for a thicker and dryer pancake, less to make thin, traditional crepes. To cook traditional crepes, pour a small amount of batter onto a small hot Teflon pan and tilt the pan aound so that the batter spreads evenly. Serve with sour cream, or protein-combatible sauce (because of the eggs) and veggies of choice.

Variation 1: add grated cheese to the batter.
Variation 2: for a sweet version, add stevia and vanilla to the batter.

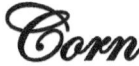

Corn

Corn Pozole
Boil large dried corn kernels with garlic, diced onion and bay leaves until soft. Serve the corn in the water it boiled in with diced onion, lemon juice, avocado, oregano, powdered hot pepper or a guajillo salsa (see Dressings and Sauces section).

Corn on the cob
Boil corn and serve with avocado (you can spread on the corn like butter), chile pepper powder and lemon. You can also substitute avocado for homemade non- hydrogenated mayonnaise, butter, sour cream and/or grated cheese.

Corn "Esquites"
Boil fresh corn cut off the cob, with sautéed onion and green salsa (optional). Add a little butter or oil at the end of the cooking time.

Variation 1: Add grated zucchini.

Oats

Oatmeal burgers
Form patties made out of soaked oatmeal, chopped onion and cilantro and brown in pan. These can also be made with sprouted whole oats that have been blended into a mush.

Cooked Vegetable Dishes

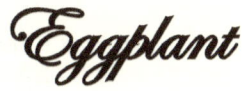

Eggplant

Eggplant in tomato sauce
Sauté or bake sliced / cubed eggplant in tomato sauce with garlic and onion.

Baba ganoush
Peel and bake eggplant in oven until soft. Blend with tahini, olive oil, roasted garlic and rosed red pepper (optional) and serve as a dip.

Marinated eggplant
Slice eggplant in thick circles and marinate in soy sauce and herbs for 2-3 hours.
Bake with other vegetables such as carrot, fennel, or zucchini in the oven,
covered with tin foil.

Eggplant pizza
Cut eggplant in thin circles and bake in a greased baking pan covered with tomato sauce and parmesan or manchego cheese.

Nopales (cactus leaves)

Nopales asados
Cook whole nopales in a Teflón pan until soft and both sides are an even shade of olive green. Slice in long pieces or serve whole with salsa of choice.

Pickled nopales

Mix steamed veggies with the cooked nopales and cook all together in a pot with aromatic herbs and apple cider vinager for 10 minutes and then let stand for another 10 to 15 minutes.

Nopale with sauce or as a salad

Boil nopales in water and chop into small (rectangular) pieces. Serve in guallilo salsa or serve as a warm or cold salad with finely diced tomato, onion and cilantro.

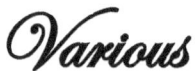

Mexican style zucchini

Finely chop and sauté zucchinis with tomato, corn and onion. Serve with avocado slices.

"Tinga" with carrot and jicama

Sauté onion and then add tomato and chipotle sauce into pan and cook until the sauce simmers. Add grated carrot and jicama and cook until soft. Serve with avocado or tofu.

Green beans

Steam grean beans until tender and then dress with olive oil, lemon juice, and oregano. Optional additions: tahini, toasted sesame seeds, soy sauce, pulverized almonds. These green beans as a side dish are favorites with all the kids, large and small.

Cauliflower and peas

Steam cauliflower florets and shelled peas together. Pan sear tomatoes and chopped onion, remove the tomato skins (they should slide off easily), discard, and mash the tomatoes with the onions.

Spoon the tomato mixture onto the vegetables and serve with sliced avocado or guacamole.

Vegetables in almond sauce
Steam your choice of vegetables (recommended: carrot, chayote, zucchini, and brocolli). To make the almond sauce, blend soaked almond with water, de-veined guajillo chiles, salt, olive oil and several pan seared tomatoes. The sauce should be thick and have a pinkish color. Pour over the vegetables in a pot or pan and continue to cook for 5-10 minutes so that the flavors combine.

Peas-in-a-pod
Steam the peas whole, in the pod, until tender. Dress with oil, soy sauce and lemon juice.or serve with a little bowl of dressing for dipping. Dip each pea pod into the dressing, then pop the whole pod into your mouth and pull out the peas with your teeth (like eating soy bean edame or artichoke leaves).

Raw or steamed vegetable salads
Chop up any raw or steamed vegetables (you can mix raw and steamed if you prefer) and serve with avocado, olive oil, lemon, soya and any salsa. Make tacos with tortillas, lettuce leaves or Nori sheets.

*Typical steamed vegetables are: green beans, chayote, zucchini, broccoli, cabbage, cauliflower, asparagus, Brussels sprouts, fennel, chives, carrots and peas.

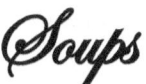

Soups

Creamy soups
Blend steamed vegetable with soaked raw soaked nuts, shelled sunflower seeds or avocado, and a little of the steaming water, salt and chile peppers or garlic (optional). Steamed chayote blended

with almonds, a touch of sea salt and roasted garlic, and chunks of browned tofu (not blended) is a favorite.

Vegetable soup
Finely chop and steam carrots, chayote, celery, peas, brócoli and cabbage in that order so the vegetables tht take longer to steam go into the pot first. Start boiling the steaming water before you start cutting the vegetables and add the vegetbles to the pot as you go. Blend enough raw tomatoes, onion, garlic, chipotle pepper (optional) and herbs of choice to cover the vegetables in the pot. Finely chop zucchini and greens such as cilantro. Once the vegetables are half way cooked, add them to the sauce and boil together for 15 minutes. Turn off the soup, add the zucchini and greens, and cover the pot for 10 minutes so the zucchini cooks in the hot broth.

Vegetable and grain soup
Same as the above soup, with the addition of your grain of choice, such as rice, wheat berries, barley, or quinoa.

Vegetable potato soup
Same as the standard vegetable soup, with the addition of cubed potatoes.

Corn and zucchini soup
Sautee onion and tomatoes, then add corn (cut off the cob) grated zuchinni and
cilantro.
Serve with sour cream or avocado.

Borsht
Saute sliced onions in a pot. Add water, shredded beets and carrots. Blend tomatoes and garlic and add to the pot. Cook until the shredded beet and carrots are soft. Serve with avocado or sour cream.

Carrot and sunflower soup

Cook shredded carrot in a little water until soft. Add a sauce of blended sunflower seed, water, cumin and soy sauce and continue cooking until sauce begins to simmer.

Cream of mushroom soup

Saute a a good deal of mushrooms (as they diminish in size when cooked) and onions together, and pan sear or steam tomatoes and a little celery. Blend the tomatoes and celery together with a little sour cream or oil and ½ of the mushrooms and onion. Add the remaining mushrooms and onion and serve with sour cream on top and parsley.

Tomato tofu soup

See Tofu, Protein section.

Chayote almond soup

See Tofu, Protein section.

Miso Soup

See Tofu, Protein section.

Raw Food
Main Dishes and Soups

Mushrooms

*Mushrooms can be substituted with zucchini or eggplant in any of the following recipes.

Barbecued mushrooms
Heat water with salt, about 1 lb of mushrooms, cover and steep till bland and then strain. Blend 3 soaked pasilla peppers, 3 soaked ancho peppers, 3 soaked mulatto peppers, ¼ cup soaked almonds, 3 soaked dates, 1 tbs vineger, 1 pinch orégano, 1 tbs carob, ¼ of 1 diced onion, 1 pinch cumin, 1 clove garlic, 1 crushed clove, 2 tbs olive oil, soy sauce and water. Add the mushrooms to the sauce and serve.

Mushrooms in green sauce
Heat water with salt, about 1 lb of mushrooms, cover and steep till bland and then strain. Blend ½ lb ground green pumpkin sedes, 8 green tomatoes, 3 serrano peppers, 1 cup of chopped cilantro, ¼ cup chopped wormwood (epazote), 2 chilaca peppers, 4 lettuce leaves, 1 garlic clove, ¼ of an onion, 1 pinch of cumin, 2 tbs olive oil, soy sauce and water. Add mushrooms to the sauce.

Mushroom Ceviche
Finely dice 1 lb of mushrooms, 8 tomatoes, 1 onion, 1 sprig cilantro, 1 serrano pepper and mix. Stir in lemon juice, soy sauce, olive oil, orégano and pieces of Nori (seaweed sheets).

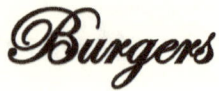

Burgers

Chickpea burgers
Blend sprouted garbanzos, onion, sesame sedes, sunflower sedes, kelp powder, garlic, parsley, cumin, lemon juice and a little water in food processor. Form into patties and dehydrate at 100 degrees for 3 hours, flip and dehydrate for another 3 hours.

Carrot burgers
Blend pulp from carrot or beet juice with the equal amount of soaked almonds, diced onion, miso, fresh herbs (parsley, dill or basil). Form into patties and dehydrate at 100 degrees for 3 hours, flip and dehydrate for another 3 hours.

Veggie burgers
Finely chop ½ cup shallots, ¾ cup spinach, ¼ cup arugula, ¼ cup tatsoy, ¼ cup celery, 1/3 cup red pepper, 1/3 cup beet, 1 tbs parsley, 1 tbs basil, 2 tbs dried orégano, 1 ½ cup mushrooms, 1 cup sun-dried tomatoes, ½ clove garlic, soy sauce in food processor. Form into patties and dehydrate at 100 degrees for 8 hours.

Mushroom burgers
Blend 1 cup of chopped mushrooms, 1 ½ cup soaked almonds, 2 carrots, 1 cup pecans, 1 serrano pepper, ½ diced onion, 2 tbs miso, 2 tbs parsley, ½ tbs orégano, 1 tsp dill and water in food processor. Form into patties and dehydrate at 100 degrees for 8 hours.

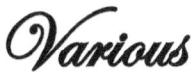
Various

Stuffed tomatoes
Dice and mix 3 stalks celery, 1 cucumber, 3 tbs soaked pine nuts, 1 cup lentil sprouts, 1 cup alfalfa sprouts and 2 tsp parsley. Cut tops off big round tomatoes, scoop out incides and fill with stuffing. Drizzle with basil dressing.

Raw Pizza
Blend about 3 cups of sprouted wheat berries, 5 tbs of flax seeds, 1 medium size onion, 2 tsp of orégano, 1 garlic clove, 2 tbs basil, 2 tbs olive oil, 2 tsp kelp powder and 2 tsp parsley in a food processor. Form into médium size round crusts on a dehydrator sheet and dehydrate at 115 degrees overnight.

Once the crust is ready, cover with a thick layer of basil pesto, 1 marinated and dehydrated eggplant, red or yellow peppers and mushrooms, tomato wheels, fresh herbs and mung bean sprouts to garnish.

Quiche 1
Blend 2 cup corn, ¼ cup ground flax seed, 1/3 cup cilantro, chopped, 1 tsp ginger, 1 tsp orange juice, 1/8 cup olive oil, ½ tsp curry, 1 chili chipotle and ½ cup sun-dried tomatoes in food processor. Mix with 1 cup sliced mushrooms and 1 cup finely chopped spinach. Dehydrate in shallow pie dish at 100 degrees for 6-8 hours. Garnish with fresh tomato and pepper slices

Quiche 2
Blend 5 cups fresh corn, 1/3 cup ground flax seed, ½ cup cilantro, 1 chipotle pepper, 1 tsp ginger, 1 tsp garlic, ½ cup orange juice, ¼ cup olive oil, 1 shallot, 1 diced small red pepper, 8 finely chopped green beans, ½ cup sliced mushrooms and ½ cup sun- dried

tomatoes. Spread in shallow pie dish and dehydrate overnight at 100 degrees.

Corn fritters
Blend 2 ½ cups corn, ¼ cup ground flax seeds, ¼ cup minced cilantro,1 tsp ginger
1tsp garlic, ¼ cup orange juice, 1/8 cup olive oil and 1 soaked date in food processor. Form into patties and dehydrate 7 hours on 100 degrees.

Seed cheese
Blend 2 cup soaked sunflower seeds, 1 tsp miso, 1 yellow bell pepper and ½ tsp curry.

Almond pate
Blend 1 ¾ cup soaked almonds and mix with 2 grated carrots, 1 finely chopped celery stalk, ½ diced red pepper, 2 tbs parsley, 6 finely chopped spinach leaves, and soy sauce.

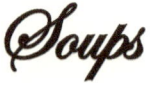

Soups

Barley vegetable
Heat water to near simmer and add 2 tbs miso, 7 grated carrots, 6 diced tomatoes, 1 minced jalepeno pepper, 1/3 cup diced red onion, 1-2 small diced shallots, 1 ½ cups of soaked barley or kamut, then turn off the heat and let sit for 5 minutes, covered.

Mexican green soup
Juice 3 celery stalks, 1 lb of green tomatoes and 3 cups of carrot juice. Blend with 1 avocado, 4 tsp cilantro and ¼ jalapeno pepper

Chunky vegetable soup

Juice 3 cups carrot juice and 6 celery stalks and blend with 1 ½ avocados and the juice of 2 lemons. Mix with 1 grated zucchini, 1 grated carrot, ¼ cup grated broccoli florets, ½ cup finely chopped arugula and 2 finely chopped celery stalks.

Avocado spinach soup

Blend 1 large avocado, 1 ½ cups spinach, ½ cup sun-dried tomatoes, the juice of 2 lemons, 2 tbs cilantro, ¼ clove garlic and 2 cups of water

Creamy corn soup

Blend ½ cup sun-dried tomatoes, 2 tsp cilantro, 1 cup corn, ½ celery stalk, ½ red pepper, 1 avocado, 1 shallot, 1 tsp miso and water.

Dressings and Salsas

Dressing

Sunflower mayo
Blend:
1 cup soaked sunflower seeds
¼ cup olive oil
1 lemon
1 tbs apple cider vinegar
1 tbs honey
½ tbs paprika
1 tbs mustard Maile
soy sauce
1 clove garlic
water

Basil cashew dressing
Blend:
¼ cup olive oil
2 cups fresh basil
1 clove garlic
1 red pepper
½ chili ancho soaked
1 cup cashews
soy sauce
water

Thousand Island dressing
Blend:
½ cup lemon juice or apple cider vinegar
¼ cup olive oil
¼ cup soaked sunflower seeds
1 red pepper
1 clove garlic
tiny piece onion

tiny piece of celery
soy sauce

Non-dairy seed sour cream
Blend:
1/3 cup dry ground sesame
2 cups soaked sunflower seeds
3 tsp olive oil
lemon
water, as necessary

Non-dairy avocado sour cream
Blend:
avocado
lemon juice to taste
sea salt

Avocado dressing
Blend:
2 lg avocados
1 sprig cilantro
1 small serrano pepper
2 tbs lemon juice
2 tbs olive oil
water
soy sauce

Basic herb dressing
Blend:
2 tbs lemon juice
½ cup olive oil
1 clove garlic
any herb of choice (cilantro, oregano, basil, parsley, thyme, sage)

Sweet and sour nut dressing
Blend:
1 cup of almonds
½ cup orange juice
½ cup lemon juice
water

Ginger dressing
Blend:
2 tsp ginger
1 tsp bragg
1 cup water
1 tbs. apple cider vinegar
1 ½ tbs olive oil

Sun-dried tomato dressing
Blend:
½ cup sun-dried tomatoes
2 lemons
1/3 of a jalepeno chili
1 tbs miso
pinch cumin seed
¾ cup water
1 tbs olive oil

Hot tahini dressing
Blend:
Tahini
Soaked chili ancho or chipotle peppers
Olive oil
Garlic
Roasted red pepper
Honey
Water
Soy sauce

Vegetable dressing
Blend:
1 tsp dried basil
1 carrot
¼ jalepeno chili
¼ red pepper
½ orange
1 tsp soy sauce
1tsp onion
1 tsp olive oil
¾ cup water

Sunflower dressing
Blend:
2 tsp sunflower seeds
¼ clove garlic
½ tsp miso
½ soy sauce
1 lemon
¼ red pepper
1 cup water

Mint dressing
Blend:
2 tbs fresh mint
2 tbs soaked sunflower seeds
¼ cup cucumber
1 lemon
1tsp soy sauce
1 cup water

Tomato-carrot quick dressing
Blend:
Carrots, tomatoes, oil, water and salt to taste. Optional: dash of lemon juice

Sweet tomato dressing
Blend:
3 lg tomatoes
1 cup sun-dried tomatoes
¼ cup basil
1 clove garlic
1 soaked date
2 tbs olive oil
1 cup water

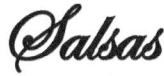

Green Salsa
Pan sear tomatillos, garlic or onion and a serrano chile and blend
with fresh cilantro. This salsa can also be made with raw tomatillos
and/or with chile de arbol.

Avocado green sauce
Blend:
1 lb fresh green tomatoes
sprig cilantro
½ clove garlic
1 jalepeno pepper
1 avocado
sea salt

Mexican red salsa
Pan seared tomatoes with garlic or onion and chile of choice and
blend all.

Guajillo salsa

Soak, de-vein and blend guajillo chiles with a little olive oil, garlic and salt.

Tomato sauce

Blend fresh or roasted:
red or green tomatoes
peppers (jalepeno, serrano, chipotle, guallilo, ancho, pasilla, arbol)
garlic, onion
(optional – oil, salt, cilantro or herbs)

Barbecue sauce 1

Blend:
Soaked chile mulato and ancho
dates
garlic
water
(optional – tomato)

Barbecue sauce 2

Blend:
5 soaked and de-seeded guallilo peppers
3 soaked and de-seeded ancho peppers
1 chile de arbol pepper
orange juice to blend
1 clove of roasted garlic
1 roasted red pepper
3 tomatoes
pinch of cumin powder

Dehydrated Breads and Crackers

Bread

* Always dehydrate at 105 degrees

Almond bread
Mix 3 cups of almond pulp, 1 cup dry ground flax seeds, 2 blended tomatoes black pepper, cumin, salt and 2 tbs olive oil. Form into loaves, cut into slices and dehydrate until firm and dry on the outside.

Thick seed bread
Ingredients:
2 cups soaked sunflower seeds
2 cups soaked pumpkin seeds
½ cup pecans
olive oil
1 cup dry ground flax
Choose and 1 of these:
Parsley
Basil
Cilantro
Dill
Thyme
Oregano

Add any of these vegetables:
Carrot
Zucchini
Tomato
Red pepper
Onion

Blend pecans in food processor. Blend soaked seeds separately. Chop vegetables and herbs, blend tomatoes and mix all ingredients. Form into loaves, slice, lie slices on the dehydrator sheets and dehydrate at 145 degrees for 1 ½ hours, flip and continue to dehydrtae for another 1 ½ hours.

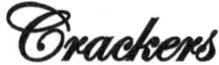

*Always dehydrate at 105 degrees.

Jicama, carrot flax crackers
Blend 4 carrots, 3 tomatoes, 4 tsp olive oil and 1 tsp tumeric in blender. Blend 2 large jicamas and 6 carrots in food processor. Mix all ingredients, add herbs, 1 lb of ground flax seeds and dehydrate overnight.

Rye crackers
Blend 2 cups sprouted rye berries, 1 cup soaked sesame seeds, ½ onion, soy sauce or sea salt, poppy seeds in food processor. Form into crackers and dehydrate overnight.

Almond crackers
Blend 1 lb soaked almonds, 6 tomatoes, 1 clove garlic, 1tbs miso in food processor and dehydrate overnight.

Sesame sunflower crackers
Blend 2 cups sprouted sunflower seeds, 2 cups sprouted sesame seeds, 1 clove garlic, 1 small piece of onion and 2 tbs miso in food processor. Add water if necessary. Dehydrate overnight.

Crispy sesame
Blend 3 cups soaked sesame seeds, 3 tomatoes, ½ red pepper, ½ clove garlic, 1 small piece of onion, soy sauce or kelp powder in food processor and dehydrate overnight.

Guajillo sesame

Same as above with the addition of soaked, de-veined and blended guajillo chiles

Miso crackers

Similar to the crispy sesame crackers recipe except for the following changes: add 2-3tbs. of miso paste, substitute soaked sunflower seeds for 1/3 of the sesame seeds and omit the 3 tomatoes.

Sweets and Treats

Cookies

*All cookies: Blend all ingredients in food processor and dehydrate overnight at 105 degrees.

Sesame banana cookies
Ingredients:
5 cup soaked sesame seeds
5 soaked dates
3 ripe bananas
1 cup raisins
1 tsp cinnamon
1 tbs vanilla

Carob banana cookies
Ingredients:
3 cups buckwheat
4 ripe bananas
½ cup soaked walnuts
1 tbs carob powder
1 tbs raw honey

Pina colada cookies
Ingredients:
pulp of 5 coconuts
2 slices of pineapple
coconut water
1 tbs honey

Apple walnut
Ingredients:
½ cup white raisins
1 cup shredded apple
½ cup walnuts, chopped

2 cups soaked wheat berries
1tsp cinnamon
2 tbs honey
Blend wheat berries, honey and water in food processor. Add remaining ingredients and mix.

Apricot
Ingredients:
½ cup walnuts, chopped
2 cup sprouted rye berries
½ cup white raisins
1 tbs Jamaican allspice
orange juice to blend
1 cup soaked apricots

Coconut cookies
Mix grated coconut with honey and vanilla. Form into balls or cookies and dehydrate overnight or freeze.

Coconut chocolate
Ingredients:
Pulp of 2 coconuts
1 cup soaked almonds
2 tbs honey
1 tsp vanilla
1 tsp carob powder

Soy fiber cookies
Mix soy fiber (well strained from soy milk), vanilla, orange or apple juice, cinamon, raisins, and carob until you have a dough-like texture. Form into cookies and freeze or dehydrate.

Tahini cherry cookies
Ingredients:
1 liter tahini
1 lb puffed amaranth

vanilla
honey
cherries
Combine ingredients and serve cold.

Raw Cakes and Pies

Piecrust 1
Blend 3 cups ground flax sedes, ½ cup soaked prunes, 1 cup soaked almonds, 1 tsp vanilla and 1 tsp orange rind in a food processor.

Piecrust 2
Blend ½ cup soaked dates, 5 cups soaked almonds or raw pecans and 1 tsp orange rind in a food processor.

Carrot cake
Blend 1 cup soaked dates, 2 cups coconut pulp, 1 piece ginger and ½ cup carrot juice in food processor. Add carrot pulp, 1 ½ cups of walnuts, cinnamon, Janaican all spice and the rinds of 3 lemons. Blend 1 ½ cups of walnuts, orange juice and vanilla separately for the frosting. Shape into cake and frost.

Coconut ice cream cake
Make pie crust 2 (refer to recipe). Blend 2 coconuts with 2 mangos, 2 bananas and vanilla. Top with stawberries and freeze.

Sesame cake
Mix toasted sesame seeds with honey and tahini. Form into a cake and freeze.

Peach cobbler

Slice 4 lbs of peaches, marinate in orange juice and honey overnight. Blend 1 ½ cups of dates, 2 ½ cups of walnuts or peacans and vanilla in food processor and form into pie crust. Top the crust the peaches and chopped nuts.

Flax zapote pie

Make a smooth layer of ground flax for the base. Mix 1 cup of tahini, 2 tbs of honey and vanilla in a bowl, add as second layer. Blend or mix zapote with orange juice as third layer. Garnish with sliced strawberries.

Ice creams

Fruit sorbet

Peel and cut any fruit into small pieces, freeze, let thaw a little and blend in a food processor. Add honey (while blending) if using slightly sour fruits and add nuts or seeds while blending if you want crunchy shorbet.

Chocolate

Blend:
½ cup soaked sunflower seeds
½ cup soaked sesame seeds
½ cup macademia nuts
½ cup soaked almonds
2 tbs honey 1 tbs carob or stawberries
1 tbs vanilla

Chocolate fudge ice cream

Blend avocados, carob, honey and vanilla until smooth. Add carob until the blended avocado looks like chocolate. Serve as chocolate pudding or freeze to make fudge ice cream.

Banana chocolate layer cake
Blend bananas with vanilla. Make a batch of fudge ice cream (refer to recipe) and por layers of each ice cream into a plastic container. Freeze, flip and remove from container.

Mango mousse
Blend:
frozen mangos
orange juice

Fig nut cream
Blend:
frozen figs
almonds
 vanilla

Banana almond
Blend:
frozen bananas
peacan
almonds
vanilla

Creamy ice cream
Blend:
any nut butter
carob
orange juice

Coconut dream
Blend:
soft coconut pulp
vanilla
cinnamon
honey

Peach mango mix
Blend:
 2 cups frozen peaches
½ cup frozen mango
1 cup soaked sunflower seeds
honey
mandarine juice
1 tbs vanilla
juice of 2 lemons

Power bars

*Blend all ingredientes, form into balls or bars and freeze or dehydrate at 105 degrees overnight.

Brownies
Blend:
½ cup soaked almonds
½ cup soaked hazelnuts
½ cup soaked sunflower seeds
½ cup soaked sesame seeds
2 tbs carob
3 tbs honey
1 tsp cinnamon

Banana date
Blend:
1 cup sprouted wheat berries
1 cup soaked almonds
3 ripe bananas
1 cup figs
1 cup soaked dates

2 tbs honey
1 tbs vanilla
1 tsp cinnamon

Chocolate hazelnut
Blend:
½ lb soaked
2 tbs carob
4 tbs honey
1 tsp vanilla
orange juice

Banana fig
Blend:
1 cup almond pulp
10 figs
3 soaked dates
2 ripe bananas
1 tbs vanilla
½ cup orange juice

Gingerbread
Blend:
4 carrots
1 med size piece ginger
4 soaked dates
½ cup soaked yellow raisins
1 tbs vanilla
¼ cup orange juice
1 tsp cinnamon

Chocolate
Blend:
nuts / toasted seeds
tahini
honey

carob
vanilla
spirulina

Coconut
Blend:
1 cup shredded coconut
1 cup soaked chopped walnuts
1 tbs raw almond butter
1 tbs carob, 2 tbs honey
1 tbs vanilla

Peanut butter
Blend:
3 tbs peanut butter
½ cup chopped walnuts
1 tbs carob
1tbs honey

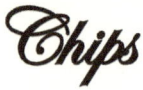

Banana chips
Slice thin strips of bananas, dehydrate at 105 degrees for 18 hours

Apple Chips
Slice thin strips of apple, sprinkle with cinnamon and stevia (optional) and dehydrate at 105 degrees overnight.

Zucchini chips
Slice zucchinis, marinate in soy sauce, olive oil, onion, garlic and chayenne pepper powder and lemon juice. Dehydrate at 105 degrees overnight.

Potato crisps

Slice potatoes into long thin strips with peeler. Marinate in soy sauce, olive oil, onion, garlic and chayenne pepper powder and lemon juice, Dehydrate at 105 degrees for 12 hours or until crisp.

Various Raw treats

Seed pudding

Blend soaked sunflower sedes, nuts and raisins or dates with hot water, add vanilla, cinnamon and grated apple or sliced banana.

Dehydrated fruit roll ups

Blend any seasonal fruit (with honey if tart) and spread on dehydrating sheets and dehydrate overnight on 105 degrees.

Raw apple raisin pancakes

Blend 4 apples, 2 cups of sprouted barley, ½ cup soaked sunflower seeds, ½ cup yellow raisins, ½ cup black raspberries, 2 tsp cinnamon, 2 tbs vanilla, 1 tbs olive oil and ¼ cup orange juice. Form into "pancakes". Dehydrate at 105 degrees.

Blackberry Fruities

Blend:
2 cup soaked sesame seeds
2 cups soaked sunflower seeds
orange juice
1 cup black raspberries
1 tsp finely grated orange rind
honey
Dehydrate overnight.

Fruit salad 1
Prepare a fruit salad (mango, papaya, grapes, banana, strawberries etc.) Blend ripe bananas with soaked almonds and vanilla or belnd natural yogurt with honey. Pour over fruit salad and serve.

Fruit salad 2
Prepare a fruit salad (mango, papaya, grapes, banana, strawberries etc.) Mix with toasted green pumkin seeds, amarinth, honey and a little orange juice.

Carob covered almonds
Mix carob, honey, vanilla and pour over unsoaked almonds. Freeze for 1 hour or more.

Green juice popsicles
Blend any greens (parsley, alfalfa, spinach, chaya) with honey / stevia and lemon, strain and freeze in popsicle trays..

Spicy Pumpkin seeds
Marinate raw pumpkin seeds in soy sauce and chile pepper powder oe cayenne powder and dehydrate overnight. Optional: add lemon juice.

Chocolate covered strawberries
Blend hazelnuts, honey, orange juice, carob, olive oil and vanilla. Dip in the strawberries and refrigerate or eat immediately.

Various Cooked treats

Oatmeal cereal
Boil oatmeal without stirring for 10 minutes. Add honey, vanilla, soaked raisins and cinnamon.

Warm corn pudding
Blend corn with water and cinnamon until smooth and creamy. Cook for 10 minutes, stirring constantly until thickened. Add honey and serve.

Pancakes with fruit dressing
Beat 2 cups of wheat or soy flour, 1 egg and ½ cup of soymilk / milk and cook pancakes on low heat in nonstick fry pan. Serve with blended stewed fruit or warm honey and butter as syrup.

Healthy popcorn
Pop dried small corn kernels in an airpopper or in a covered pan / pot over low heat. Move the pan / pot in a circular motion as the kernels start popping to avoid burning. Continue moving the pot until the popping stops. Add butter, / olive oil and salt.

Carob (soy) milk
Soak 1 cup soy beans overnight. Heat beans to a near boil. Blend in (powerful blender such as a Vitamix) with 2 liters water and strain. Save the soy fiber to make cookies! Add honey, carob and vanilla to soy milk.

An Important Note To Readers
June 2014

Dear Readers,
Recently I was introduced to Dr. Graham's 80-10-10 diet. I need to express how fully I endorse it as a Chakra 5 and 6 diet, if that is appropriate for your current life lessons. All of my nutrition books can be used as a transition to Dr. Graham's diet, which is a pure Chakra 5 & 6 diet. The more greens and non-sweet vegetables one consumes, the more it is a Chakra 5 diet. The more sweet fruit, the more it would fall into a Ch. 6 diet category.

All of the nutrition knowledge in my books must therefore please be modified, reducing the fat intake to achieve an 80-10-10 ratio ideally or no more than 30% fat initially as you are reducing. As raw foodists, we have all erroneously over-consumed very high fat foods such as cold-pressed olive oil, nuts and seeds and avocados. To give you an idea: if you consume approximately 2000 calories a day, ideally you should not consume more than 100g of an avocado a day (a third of a medium to large avocado), OR the equivalent of 15 almonds, OR 1 tbs. of olive oil. If you raise your caloric intake, then you would be able to eat more fat and more protein. The important thing is that your ratio approximates the ideal 80-10-10. You can accumulate these quantities - eat no fat for a three days and then eat an avocado in the evening with your salad.

There is a very simple website – www.nutridiary.com – that calculates the percentages of your daily caloric food intake. I really advise you to get someone to teach you the basics of how to use the site, which would take no more than a half an hour class at the most. If you don't know anyone to teach it to you, Tashirat can send you an instruction video. Write us your request to the email listed at our website: (www.tashirat.com).

If you find it too challenging to transition to the 80-10-10 diet alone, we can help you with consultations in person or by e-mail. Just contact us and we'll gladly help you. We also offer nutrition courses, which include Yoga, Meditation and Chakra classes.

To conclude, anyone interested in nutrition needs to read Dr. Graham's outstandingly simple, clear and informative 80-10-10 book. I wish I would have found it 30 years ago but the book only came out in 2008 and I was only introduced to it very recently. I'm in 100% agreement with all that he so eloquently and concisely imparts in his valuable book. One cannot expect emotional, mental and spiritual body health and happiness (balance), without achieving physical body health.

Dr. Graham's book has to be supplemented by all of my nutrition books, which are essential as they focus on vibrational nutrition.

To Health, Love and Life!

With love,
Artimia

p.s. I do not personally know Dr. Douglas Graham, but from over a year of experience on ourselves, our Tashirat children and students we find the 80/10/10 diet that Dr. Graham promotes invaluable as a Chakra 5 & 6 diet.

If transitioned correctly, fully taking into consideration the person's vibration, evolution and present physical condition, the 80/10/10 diet is excellent information.